DISCLAIMER

The information in this book is not intended as medical advice. The content is for information and research purposes only.

By reading this disclaimer, you fully accept the terms of this disclaimer. If you are not in agreement with this disclaimer, please do not order or read this book. The content of this book is provided for information and educational purposes only. Kindly do not interpret this book or its content for a medication or product. This is only a book guide.

Thanks

4

INTRODUCTION

Explanation of Boron

Are you tired of constantly battling with diseases and inflammation? Have you tried countless remedies with no success? Look no further than Boron. This miracle element that has been hiding in plain sight has been found to have a significant impact on human health. From boosting bone health to alleviating menopausal symptoms, Boron has been proven to be a natural remedy for a variety of health concerns. In this book, we will explore the research behind Boron and its ability to cure all diseases and inflammation.

For centuries, Boron has been used for various purposes. It was first discovered in the Middle East, where it was used in the production of glass and ceramics. It wasn't until the 20th century that scientists began to study the impact of Boron on human health. As research progressed, it became clear that Boron was much more than just a useful element for industrial purposes.

Boron has been found to have many benefits for human health. For starters, it is essential for bone health. Boron has been proven to increase bone density and reduce the risk of osteoporosis. It also plays a crucial role in regulating hormones, particularly testosterone and estrogen. This makes it an effective natural remedy for hormone-related health concerns such as menopause and low libido.

In addition to its impact on bone health and hormone regulation, Boron has also been found to have anti-inflammatory properties. Chronic inflammation is linked to a variety of health concerns, including arthritis, inflammatory bowel disease, and allergies. Boron can help reduce chronic inflammation and alleviate these health concerns.

Boron has also been found to have a significant impact on brain function. Research has shown that it can improve cognitive function and memory, making it an effective natural remedy for attention deficit hyperactivity disorder (ADHD) and other brain-related health concerns.

Despite its many benefits, Boron is not widely known or used. Many people are unaware of its ability to cure all diseases and inflammation. This is why we have written this book, to shed light on the incredible benefits of Boron and to provide a comprehensive guide to its usage.

Throughout this book, we will delve deeper into the research behind Boron and its impact on various health concerns. We will explore the different food sources of Boron and the dosages that are recommended for optimal health benefits. We will also discuss Boron supplements and how they can be used to improve health.

We will focus on the role of Boron in bone health and hormone regulation, exploring the ways in which it can be used as a natural remedy for these health concerns. We will also explore the impact of Boron on inflammation and brain function, discussing the research that has been conducted on these topics.

In addition, we will discuss the impact of Boron on menopausal symptoms, providing insights into how it can alleviate hot flashes, vaginal dryness, and mood swings.

By the end of this book, you will have a thorough understanding of the incredible benefits of Boron and how it can be used as a natural remedy for all diseases and inflammation. We hope that this book will inspire you to take advantage of the miracle of Boron and to experience the benefits for themselves. Say goodbye to your health worries and say hello to the power of Boron.

Brief history of Boron

Boron has a long and fascinating history, with its origins dating back to the Middle East. It was first discovered in the form of borax, a white crystalline mineral that was used for a variety of purposes, including the production of glass and ceramics.

The first recorded use of borax dates back to the 9th century, when it was used by Arab goldsmiths as a flux for soldering gold and silver. It was also used in medicine, with Arab physicians using it to treat eye infections and wounds.

In the 17th century, European chemists began to study borax and its properties. The German chemist Wilhelm Homberg was the first to isolate boron in 1702, although he did not realize what he had discovered at the time.

It wasn't until the 1800s that boron was identified as an element. In 1808, the French chemist Joseph Louis Gay-Lussac and the British chemist Humphry Davy independently produced small amounts of boron by heating boron oxide with potassium. They both observed the formation of a brown powder, which they later identified as a new element.

Over the years, boron continued to be studied and its properties were explored. In the early 20th century, scientists began to investigate the potential health benefits of boron. One of the earliest studies was conducted by Dr. Francis Pottenger, who was interested in the impact of boron on bone health.

Dr. Pottenger conducted a study on the effects of boron on the bones of chickens. He found that the chickens who were given a boron-deficient diet had weaker bones and were more likely to develop arthritis. This led him to conclude that boron was essential for bone health.

Further research was conducted in the following decades, with scientists exploring the impact of boron on hormone regulation, brain function, and inflammation. The results were promising, with boron showing significant potential as a natural remedy for a variety of health concerns.

One of the key ways in which boron has been found to cure diseases is through its impact on bone health. Boron is essential for the development and maintenance of strong bones, and it has been found to increase bone density and reduce the risk of osteoporosis.

Boron has also been found to play a crucial role in hormone regulation. It can help to balance testosterone and estrogen levels, making it an effective natural remedy for hormone-related health concerns such as menopause and low libido.

In addition to its impact on bone health and hormone regulation, boron has been found to have anti-inflammatory properties. Chronic inflammation is linked to a variety of health concerns, including arthritis, inflammatory bowel disease, and allergies. Boron can help reduce chronic inflammation and alleviate these health concerns.

Boron has also been found to have a significant impact on brain function. Research has shown that it can improve cognitive function and memory, making it an effective natural remedy for attention deficit hyperactivity disorder (ADHD) and other brain-related health concerns.

Today, boron is used in a variety of forms, including boron supplements and boron-rich foods. While more research is needed to fully understand the potential health benefits of boron, there is no doubt that it has significant potential as a natural remedy for all diseases and inflammation.

Why and where is boron banned?

While boron has been found to have significant potential as a natural remedy for a variety of health concerns, it is partially banned for use in some parts of the world due to concerns about its safety.

In the European Union, the use of boron in cosmetics is restricted to a maximum concentration of 0.2%. This is due to concerns about the potential for boron to accumulate in the body and cause toxicity.

In the United States, boron is classified as a dietary supplement and is available over-the-counter. However, the Food and Drug Administration (FDA) has not approved any health claims for boron supplements, and there is a lack of consensus among health experts about the appropriate dosage for boron.

In Australia, the use of boron in cosmetics is prohibited due to concerns about its potential toxicity. However, it is still used in a variety of other products, including cleaning agents and pesticides.

Boron is also banned for use in agriculture in some parts of the world. In India, the use of boron as a soil additive is banned due to concerns about its potential toxicity to crops and the environment. In the European Union, the use of boron as a fertilizer is restricted to a maximum concentration of 2%.

While the partial bans on boron usage around the world may be a cause for concern, it is important to note that these restrictions are primarily aimed at preventing overexposure to the substance. When used in moderation and according to recommended guidelines, boron supplements and other boron-containing products are generally considered safe.

It is also worth noting that boron occurs naturally in many foods, including fruits, vegetables, and nuts. As such, it is unlikely that individuals who consume a varied and balanced diet will experience any adverse effects from boron exposure.

In conclusion, while boron is partially banned for use in some parts of the world, it remains a promising natural remedy for a variety of health concerns. As with any supplement or medication, it is important to follow recommended guidelines and consult with a healthcare provider before using boron products.

Latest applications for boron/borax

Boron and borax continue to have a wide range of applications in various industries. Here are some of the latest and most notable applications:

- **Energy storage:** Boron-based materials have been found to have potential applications in energy storage, particularly in the development of high-capacity batteries. Researchers are investigating the use of boron-doped graphene as an electrode material in lithium-ion batteries.

- **Nuclear energy:** Boron is used as a neutron absorber in nuclear reactors. In particular, boron carbide has been found to be an effective material for controlling nuclear reactions and for use in radiation shielding.

- **Aerospace:** Boron fibers and composites are used in the aerospace industry to produce lightweight, high-strength materials for aircraft and spacecraft structures. Boron fibers are also used in the production of rocket nozzles.

- **Agriculture:** Boron is an essential micronutrient for plant growth, and is used as a fertilizer to improve crop yields. Boron is also used as a pesticide in the form of boric acid, which is effective against a range of insects and pests.

- **Glass and ceramics:** Boron compounds are used in the production of high-strength glass and ceramics. Borosilicate glass, for example, is used in laboratory glassware, optical components, and cookware due to its high resistance to thermal shock.

- **Health and wellness:** Boron supplements continue to gain popularity as a natural remedy for a range of health concerns, including arthritis, osteoporosis, and cognitive decline.

Boron supplements are also marketed as a testosterone booster, although the evidence for this claim is limited.

- **Water treatment:** Boron compounds are used in water treatment to remove impurities and contaminants. Borax, for example, is used in swimming pools and spas to regulate pH levels and prevent the growth of algae.

These are just a few of the latest applications for boron and borax. As research into the properties and potential applications of boron continues, it is likely that even more innovative uses will be discovered.

Importance of Boron for human health

Boron is an essential trace element that is crucial for maintaining good health. While boron is not classified as a traditional mineral, it plays a vital role in a number of physiological processes. Here are some of the key ways in which boron is important for human health:

- **Bone health:** Boron is essential for maintaining healthy bones. It works in conjunction with calcium, magnesium, and vitamin D to promote bone mineralization and prevent bone loss. Studies have shown that boron supplementation can improve bone density in postmenopausal women and individuals with osteoarthritis.

- **Joint health:** Boron has anti-inflammatory properties that make it useful for reducing joint pain and stiffness. It is particularly effective for individuals with rheumatoid arthritis, where it has been shown to reduce pain, swelling, and morning stiffness.

- **Brain function:** Boron plays a role in cognitive function and may have a protective effect against cognitive decline. Studies have shown that boron supplementation can improve memory, attention, and hand-eye coordination in healthy adults.

- **Hormonal health:** Boron is involved in the production and metabolism of hormones, including estrogen and testosterone. Studies have shown that boron supplementation can increase testosterone levels in men, which may have a positive impact on muscle mass, bone density, and cognitive function.

- **Wound healing:** Boron has been found to promote wound healing by increasing the production of collagen, a protein that is essential for tissue repair.

- **Metabolism:** Boron is involved in a number of metabolic processes, including carbohydrate metabolism and the regulation of insulin levels. Studies have shown that boron supplementation can improve glucose tolerance and insulin sensitivity in individuals with type 2 diabetes.

- **Immune function:** Boron has been found to have immune-modulating effects, meaning that it can help to regulate the immune system. It has been shown to enhance the activity of natural killer cells, which are important for fighting off infections and tumors.

Boron is a vital nutrient that is essential for maintaining good health. Its role in bone and joint health, brain function, hormonal health, wound healing, metabolism, and immune function make it an important element in the human diet. While boron deficiency is rare, ensuring adequate intake through a balanced diet or supplementation may provide numerous health benefits.

Chemical structure of Boron

The chemical symbol for boron is B, and its atomic number is 5. It belongs to group 13 of the periodic table and has an electron configuration of [He] 2s2 2p1. Boron is a metalloid, meaning that it has properties of both metals and non-metals.

At the atomic level, boron has three electrons in its outer shell. This makes it unique among the elements, as it is the only element in group 13 with fewer than four valence electrons. This electron deficiency gives boron its distinctive chemical and physical properties.

The chemical structure of boron is based on its atomic structure. Boron atoms have a small atomic radius, which allows them to form strong covalent bonds with other elements. The most common form of boron is boron trioxide (B2O3), which is a white, crystalline solid that is used in the production of glass and ceramics.

In addition to its role in boron trioxide, boron also forms a wide range of other compounds, including boron carbide (B4C), boron nitride (BN), and borax (Na2B4O7•10H2O). These compounds have a range of applications in industry, medicine, and agriculture.

Overall, the unique atomic and chemical properties of boron make it an important element in a wide range of applications. Its small atomic radius, electron deficiency, and strong covalent bonding make it useful for producing high-strength materials, while its essential role in human health makes it a vital nutrient for maintaining good health.

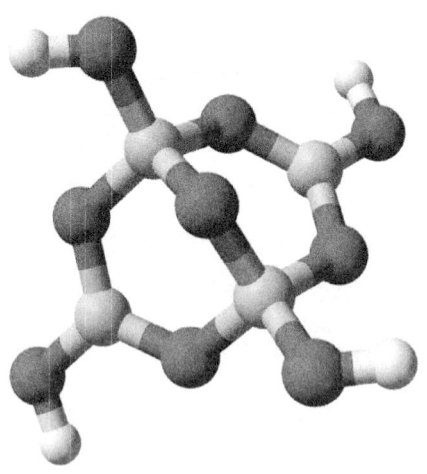

CHAPTER ONE

The Benefits of Boron

Boron is a trace element that is essential for maintaining good health. Despite its relative obscurity, boron has been discovered to have various health benefits. In this chapter, we will go over some of the most important boron advantages in greater depth.

Boosting bone health

Boron is essential for maintaining healthy bones. It works in conjunction with calcium, magnesium, and vitamin D to promote bone mineralization and prevent bone loss. Studies have shown that boron supplementation can improve bone density in postmenopausal women and individuals with osteoarthritis. Boron is also important for preventing bone fractures and reducing the risk of osteoporosis.

Regulating hormones

Boron is involved in the production and metabolism of hormones, including estrogen and testosterone. Studies have shown that boron supplementation can increase testosterone levels in men, which may have a positive impact on muscle mass, bone density, and cognitive function. Boron may also be beneficial for women, as it has been shown to reduce the symptoms of menopause.

Reducing inflammation

Boron has anti-inflammatory properties that make it useful for reducing joint pain and stiffness. It is particularly effective for individuals with rheumatoid arthritis, where it has been shown to reduce pain, swelling, and morning stiffness. Boron also has a positive effect on the immune system, which can help to prevent chronic inflammation.

Improving brain function

Boron plays a role in cognitive function and may have a protective effect against cognitive decline. Studies have shown that boron supplementation can improve memory, attention, and hand-eye coordination in healthy adults. Boron may also be beneficial for individuals with cognitive impairments, such as Alzheimer's disease.

Fighting arthritis

Boron has been found to be effective in reducing the symptoms of arthritis. It can reduce joint pain and inflammation, as well as improve mobility and flexibility. Boron is particularly useful for individuals with osteoarthritis and rheumatoid arthritis.

Alleviating menopausal symptoms

Boron has been shown to reduce the symptoms of menopause, such as hot flashes and night sweats. It may also improve bone density and prevent bone loss in postmenopausal women.

Enhancing wound healing

Boron has been found to promote wound healing by increasing the production of collagen, a protein that is essential for tissue repair. It can also reduce inflammation and pain associated with wounds.

Managing Cancer

Boron has been found to be effective in managing cancer. It has been shown to have anti-tumor properties, particularly in breast cancer and prostate cancer. Boron may also enhance the effectiveness of chemotherapy drugs.

Heart Health

Boron may improve heart health by reducing inflammation and oxidative stress, as well as regulating blood pressure and cholesterol levels. Studies have shown that boron supplementation can improve endothelial function, which is an important marker of cardiovascular health.

Boron in Pregnancy and for infants

Boron is important for fetal development and may help to prevent birth defects. It is also important for infant growth and development, particularly for bone and brain development. Pregnant women and breastfeeding mothers should ensure that they are getting adequate amounts of boron in their diet.

In conclusion, boron is a vital nutrient that offers a range of health benefits. Its role in bone and joint health, brain function, hormonal health, wound healing, cancer management, heart health, and infant development make it an important element in the human diet. While boron deficiency is rare, ensuring adequate intake through a balanced diet or supplementation may provide numerous health benefits.

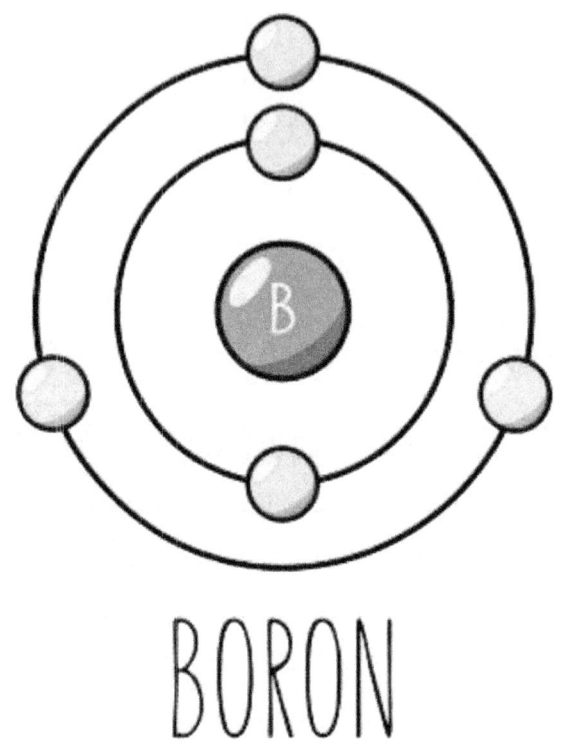

BORON

CHAPTER TWO

Sources of Boron

Food sources of Boron

Boron is a trace mineral that is found in many foods. While the daily requirement for boron is relatively low, it is important to ensure that you are getting enough of this vital nutrient in your diet. Here are some of the best food sources of boron:

Nuts and seeds

Nuts and seeds are some of the best sources of boron. Almonds, peanuts, hazelnuts, and sunflower seeds are all high in boron. You can eat these as a snack or add them to your meals for a boost of boron.

Fruits

Fruits are also a good source of boron. Apples, pears, peaches, grapes, and raisins are all high in boron. You can eat these as a snack or add them to your meals for a boost of boron.

Vegetables

Vegetables are another good source of boron. Broccoli, cauliflower, spinach, and potatoes are all high in boron. You can eat these as a side dish or add them to your meals for a boost of boron.

Legumes

Legumes, such as beans, lentils, and peas, are also a good source of boron. You can add these to your meals as a side dish or use them as a base for soups and stews.

Whole grains

Whole grains, such as brown rice and quinoa, are also a good source of boron. You can use these as a base for meals or add them to soups and stews for a boost of boron.

Meat and dairy products

Meat and dairy products are also sources of boron, although in smaller amounts compared to plant-based sources. Beef, chicken, fish, and milk are all sources of boron. It is important to choose lean sources of meat and dairy to avoid excess saturated fats and calories.

Supplements

Boron supplements are available in various forms such as capsules, tablets, powders, and liquids. They are marketed as a convenient way to increase the intake of boron for individuals who cannot meet their daily requirement through diet alone. Here are some of the different supplements of boron and how they are taken:

Boron Capsules and Tablets

Boron capsules and tablets are available in various dosages, ranging from 3mg to 20mg per serving. They are usually taken once or twice a day with water or a meal. It is important to follow the recommended dosage instructions on the packaging and consult a healthcare professional before taking any supplements to avoid any adverse effects and interactions with medications.

Boron Powder

Boron powder is also available as a dietary supplement. It is usually added to water, juice, or smoothies and taken once or twice a day. The recommended dosage of boron powder varies depending on the brand, and it is important to follow the instructions on the packaging and consult a healthcare professional before taking any supplements.

Boron Liquid

Boron liquid is another form of boron supplement that is available in various strengths. It can be added to water or juice and taken once or twice a day. The recommended dosage of boron liquid varies depending on the brand, and it is important to follow the instructions on the packaging and consult a healthcare professional before taking any supplements.

Multivitamin Supplements

Many multivitamin supplements contain small amounts of boron along with other essential vitamins and minerals. They are usually taken once a day with a meal. It is important to choose a reputable brand and follow the recommended dosage instructions on the packaging.

In conclusion, boron supplements are available in various forms, including capsules, tablets, powders, and liquids. They are marketed as a convenient way to increase the intake of boron, but it is important to consult a healthcare professional before taking any supplements to avoid any adverse effects and interactions with medications. Additionally, it is always best to try to meet your daily requirement of boron through a healthy and balanced diet.

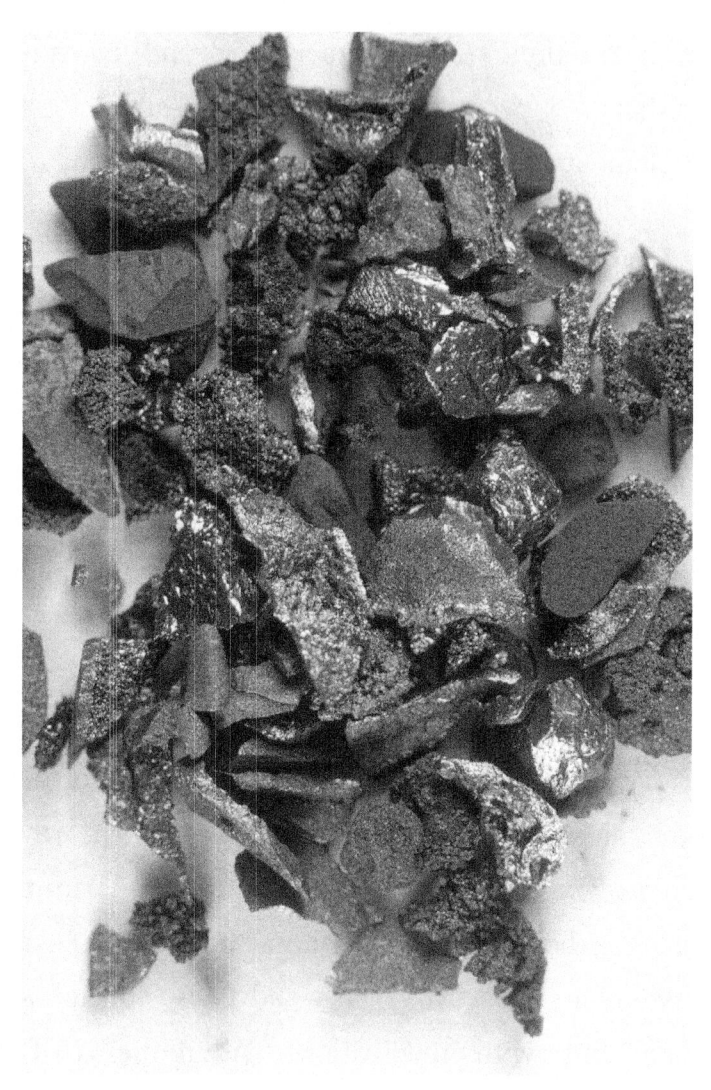

CHAPTER THREE

Boron and Bone Health

The role of Boron in bone health

Boron is a mineral that is necessary for maintaining and strengthening bone health. It works by assisting in the absorption and metabolism of calcium, magnesium, and vitamin D, all of which are necessary for bone growth and preservation. Boron aids bone health in the following ways:

Increased Calcium and Magnesium Absorption

Boron helps the body to absorb calcium and magnesium, which are essential minerals for bone health. Calcium and magnesium are the main components of bones, and without them, bones become weak and fragile. Boron enhances the absorption of these minerals by increasing the activity of enzymes that are involved in their metabolism.

Improved Vitamin D Metabolism

Boron also helps the body to utilize vitamin D more effectively. Vitamin D is necessary for calcium absorption and bone growth. Without vitamin D, the body cannot absorb calcium from the diet. Boron helps the body to convert vitamin D into an active form that can be utilized by the body.

Increased Bone Density

Studies have shown that boron supplementation can increase bone density, especially in postmenopausal women. Bone density is a measure of the amount of minerals in bones, and a higher bone density means stronger bones that are less likely to fracture.

Reduced Risk of Osteoporosis

Osteoporosis is a condition where bones become weak and fragile, increasing the risk of fractures. Boron has been shown to reduce the risk of osteoporosis by improving bone density and strength. Boron supplementation has been shown to reduce the excretion of calcium and magnesium in urine, which helps to maintain their levels in the body and prevent bone loss.

In conclusion, boron plays a crucial role in maintaining and improving bone health. It supports the absorption and metabolism of essential nutrients such as calcium, magnesium, and vitamin D, which are necessary for bone growth and maintenance. Boron supplementation has been shown to increase bone density and reduce the risk of osteoporosis. It is important to ensure adequate intake of boron through a balanced diet or supplementation to support optimal bone health.

Boron and osteoporosis

Osteoporosis is a condition characterized by low bone density and deterioration of bone tissue, leading to an increased risk of fractures. Boron plays an important role in bone health and may be helpful in preventing and treating osteoporosis. Boron helps to improve bone density by supporting the absorption and metabolism of calcium, magnesium, and vitamin D, which are essential nutrients for bone growth and maintenance. In addition, boron has been shown to increase levels of hormones that stimulate bone growth and reduce levels of hormones that contribute to bone loss.

Boron supplementation has been found in studies to increase bone density and lower the incidence of osteoporosis. One study found that postmenopausal women who took boron supplements for 6 months had significantly higher bone density than those who received a placebo. Another study discovered that boron supplementation lowered levels of a bone breakdown marker in postmenopausal women, indicating a lower risk of osteoporosis.

The recommended dosage of boron for osteoporosis prevention and treatment varies depending on the individual's age, gender, and health status. The National Institutes of Health recommends a daily intake of 1-13 mg of boron for adults, with higher doses recommended for pregnant and lactating women. Boron supplements are available in various forms, including capsules, tablets, and liquid drops. It is important to consult a healthcare provider before starting any boron supplementation to determine the appropriate dosage and ensure that it does not interact with any medications.

In conclusion, boron is essential for maintaining and improving bone health, and boron supplementation may aid in the prevention and treatment of osteoporosis. Boron aids in the absorption and metabolism of critical minerals for bone formation and maintenance, and it may boost levels of hormones that promote bone growth while decreasing levels of hormones that promote bone loss. Boron dose for osteoporosis prevention and therapy varies by individual, thus it is necessary to see a healthcare expert before beginning any supplementation.

Boron and bone fractures

Boron has been found to be beneficial in preventing and reducing the risk of bone fractures. Studies have shown that boron helps to increase bone strength, which reduces the risk of fractures, and also speeds up the healing process of broken bones. Boron works by improving the absorption and utilization of important bone-building minerals such as calcium and magnesium, which are crucial for maintaining bone strength and density.

Boron supplementation boosted bone strength and reduced the incidence of fractures in postmenopausal women, according to a study published in the Journal of Trace Elements in Medicine and Biology. Boron supplementation increased bone repair in individuals with wrist fractures, according to another study published in the Journal of Alternative and Complementary Medicine.

The recommended dosage of boron for reducing the risk of bone fractures and improving bone healing is 3-6 mg per day for adults. Higher dosages may be needed for individuals with specific health conditions or who are at a higher risk of fractures.

It is important to note that boron supplementation should be used as a complementary treatment for fractures and should not replace conventional medical treatments such as immobilization or surgery. It is also important to consult with a healthcare professional before starting any boron supplementation to ensure that it is safe and appropriate for the individual's needs.

In summary, boron has been found to be beneficial in reducing the risk of bone fractures and improving bone healing. Boron works by improving the absorption and utilization of important bone-building minerals such as calcium and magnesium. The recommended dosage of boron for reducing the risk of bone fractures and improving bone healing is 3-6 mg per day for adults, but higher dosages may be needed for individuals with specific health conditions or who are at a higher risk of fractures. It is important to consult with a healthcare professional before starting any boron supplementation to ensure that it is safe and appropriate for the individual's needs.

Boron and Hormone Regulation

Boron is a trace element that is essential for the normal growth and development of plants, animals, and humans. It is found naturally in food sources such as fruits, vegetables, nuts, and legumes. While it has many biological roles, one of the most important is its involvement in hormone regulation.

Hormones are chemical messengers that are produced by the endocrine glands and travel throughout the body to regulate various physiological functions. Boron plays a critical role in the synthesis and metabolism of certain hormones, particularly those related to bone health and reproductive function.

Boron has been shown to improve bone health, owing to its capacity to boost the levels of various hormones involved in bone metabolism. One of these hormones is estrogen, which is necessary for bone density maintenance and the prevention of osteoporosis. Boron supplementation has been demonstrated in studies to boost levels of circulating estrogen in postmenopausal women, resulting in increased bone mineral density and a lower risk of fracture.

In addition to its effects on estrogen, boron also plays a role in the regulation of other hormones related to bone health, such as vitamin D and parathyroid hormone. Vitamin D is essential for the absorption of calcium, which is crucial for bone health, and boron has been found to increase the conversion of vitamin D to its active form. Parathyroid hormone, on the other hand, regulates calcium and phosphate levels in the blood, and boron has been shown to enhance its activity.

Boron also helps to regulate reproductive hormones, including testosterone and estradiol. Male reproductive health requires testosterone, whereas female reproductive health requires estradiol. Boron has been shown to raise the levels of both hormones in the blood, resulting in increased desire and sexual performance.

Boron has also been reported to have anti-inflammatory and antioxidant properties, which may be related to its role in hormone control. Inflammation and oxidative stress are known to alter hormone balance, and boron may aid to preserve hormonal equilibrium by lowering these processes.

Boron plays an important role in hormone regulation, particularly those related to bone health and reproductive function. Its effects on estrogen, testosterone, vitamin D, and parathyroid hormone make it a promising supplement for individuals at risk for osteoporosis or sexual dysfunction. However, more research is needed to fully understand the mechanisms by which boron affects hormone balance and to determine optimal dosages for supplementation.

Boron and testosterone

Boron has been shown to have a positive effect on testosterone levels, which can improve male fertility. Testosterone is a male sex hormone that plays a crucial role in reproductive health and fertility. Low testosterone levels have been linked to infertility in men.

Studies have found that boron supplementation can increase testosterone levels in both men and women. A study found that boron supplementation increased free testosterone levels in healthy male subjects. Another study published in the journal Nutrients found that boron supplementation increased testosterone levels in men with low testosterone levels.

Boron's effect on testosterone levels is thought to be due to its ability to increase levels of sex hormone-binding globulin (SHBG), a protein that binds to testosterone and regulates its availability. By increasing SHBG levels, boron can increase the amount of testosterone that is available for use in the body.

Boron is best taken in doses of 6-10 mg per day to improve male fertility. It is vital to highlight that boron supplements should be used in conjunction with standard medical therapies for infertility. Before beginning any boron supplementation, it is also vital to consult with a healthcare expert to ensure that it is safe and appropriate for the individual's needs.

In conclusion, it has been demonstrated that boron increases testosterone levels, which can improve male fertility. Boron is considered to affect testosterone levels through increasing levels of sex hormone-binding globulin (SHBG). Boron is best taken in doses of 6-10 mg per day to improve male fertility. Boron supplementation, on the other hand, should be used as a supplemental treatment and should not be utilized in place of traditional medical treatments for infertility. Before beginning any boron supplements, it is critical to consult with a healthcare expert.

Boron and estrogen

Boron plays a role in estrogen metabolism, and studies suggest that it may have a positive effect on female fertility by improving estrogen balance. Estrogen is a female sex hormone that plays a key role in reproductive health and fertility. Imbalances in estrogen levels have been linked to fertility issues, including irregular menstrual cycles and difficulty getting pregnant.

According to research, boron may help regulate estrogen levels by boosting the enzyme aromatase, which converts androgens (male hormones) to estrogens. Boron may also aid in the increase of 17-beta-estradiol, a type of estrogen vital for female reproductive health.

Boron supplementation has been shown in studies to increase reproductive results in women. Boron supplementation enhanced menstrual regularity and hormone levels in women with polycystic ovarian syndrome (PCOS), a disorder that can lead to infertility, according to one study published in the journal Biological Trace Element Research. Another study published in the journal Environmental Health and Preventive Medicine discovered that boron supplementation enhanced reproductive outcomes in women undergoing IVF.

The recommended dosage of boron for improving female fertility is 3-10 mg per day. However, it is important to note that boron supplementation should be used as a complementary treatment and should not replace conventional medical treatments for infertility. It is also important to consult with a healthcare professional before starting any boron supplementation to ensure that it is safe and appropriate for the individual's needs.

In summary, boron may have a positive effect on female fertility by improving estrogen balance. Boron may help regulate estrogen levels by increasing levels of aromatase and 17-beta-estradiol. Studies have found that boron supplementation can improve fertility outcomes in women. The recommended dosage of boron for improving female fertility is 3-10 mg per day. However, boron supplementation should be used as a complementary treatment and should not replace conventional medical treatments for infertility. It is important to consult with a healthcare professional before starting any boron supplementation.

Boron and thyroid hormones

Vital trace mineral called boron is needed for the body to function properly. Boron may be involved in the control of thyroid hormones, according to some theories. Several crucial physiological functions, including growth and development, metabolism, and control of body temperature, are aided by the hormones produced by the thyroid gland.

According to research, boron supplementation can enhance thyroid function in those who are deficient. For instance, a study indicated that supplementing with boron improved thyroid function in individuals with low thyroid hormone levels, according to research published in the Journal of Trace Elements in Medicine and Biology. In another study that was published in the journal Environmental Health Perspectives, rats who were fed boron-deficient diets showed improved thyroid hormone levels in response to boron supplementation.

The recommended daily intake of boron for adults is 1-3 mg per day. However, the optimal dosage of boron for improving thyroid function has not been established. It is important to note that excessive boron intake can be toxic and may cause adverse effects such as nausea, vomiting, and diarrhea.

Therefore, it is recommended that individuals who wish to supplement with boron for thyroid health do so under the guidance of a healthcare professional. They can help determine the appropriate dosage based on individual needs and monitor for any potential side effects or interactions with other medications.

In summary, boron may play a role in the regulation of thyroid hormones. Research has shown that boron supplementation can improve thyroid function in people with deficiencies. However, the optimal dosage of boron for improving thyroid function has not been established. The recommended daily intake of boron for adults is 1-3 mg per day. It is recommended that individuals who wish to supplement with boron for thyroid health do so under the guidance of a healthcare professional.

Boron and Inflammation

Inflammation is a natural response of the body's immune system to infection or injury. However, chronic inflammation can contribute to the development of many diseases, including arthritis, cardiovascular disease, and cancer. Boron has been suggested to have anti-inflammatory properties, which may help reduce the risk of these diseases.

Boron may help reduce inflammation by influencing the production of cytokines, which are proteins involved in the immune response. Research has shown that boron supplementation can decrease the production of pro-inflammatory cytokines such as interleukin-1 beta (IL-1β) and tumor necrosis factor-alpha (TNF-α). In addition, boron may also help increase the production of anti-inflammatory cytokines such as interleukin-10 (IL-10).

Boron has also been suggested to have antioxidant properties, which may help reduce inflammation. Antioxidants help protect cells from damage caused by free radicals, which are unstable molecules that can cause oxidative stress and inflammation.

According to one study, postmenopausal women who took boron supplements had lower levels of C-reactive protein (CRP), a sign of inflammation. In another study, boron supplementation was found to lower inflammatory markers in rheumatoid arthritis patients, according to research appearing in the journal Bio Factors.

Adults should consume 1-3 mg of boron daily on average. The best amount of boron to use for decreasing inflammation hasn't yet been determined.

It's crucial to remember that consuming too much boron can be poisonous and result in side effects like nausea, vomiting, and diarrhea.

Therefore, it is recommended that individuals who wish to supplement with boron for reducing inflammation do so under the guidance of a healthcare professional. They can help determine the appropriate dosage based on individual needs and monitor for any potential side effects or interactions with other medications.

In summary, boron has been suggested to have anti-inflammatory properties, which may help reduce the risk of many diseases. Boron may help reduce inflammation by influencing the production of cytokines and by acting as an antioxidant. However, the optimal dosage of boron for reducing inflammation has not been established, and excessive boron intake can be toxic. Therefore, it is recommended that individuals who wish to supplement with boron for reducing inflammation do so under the guidance of a healthcare professional.

Boron and arthritis

Arthritis is a chronic inflammatory disorder that causes pain and stiffness in the joints. Boron has been shown to have anti-inflammatory qualities, which may help lessen arthritis symptoms and enhance joint health.

Boron supplementation has been demonstrated in studies to reduce inflammatory indicators in the blood, such as C-reactive protein (CRP) and erythrocyte sedimentation rate (ESR), which are typically increased in persons with arthritis. Boron may also help boost antioxidant levels in the body, which can reduce inflammation and protect joint tissues from injury.

One study published in the Journal of Trace Elements in Medicine and Biology found that boron supplementation reduced joint pain and stiffness in patients with osteoarthritis. Another study published in the Journal of Nutritional Medicine found that boron supplementation improved grip strength and reduced pain in patients with rheumatoid arthritis.

The recommended daily intake of boron for adults is 1-3 mg per day. However, the optimal dosage of boron for treating arthritis has not been established. It is important to note that excessive boron intake can be toxic and may cause adverse effects such as nausea, vomiting, and diarrhea.

Therefore, it is recommended that individuals who wish to supplement with boron for arthritis do so under the guidance of a healthcare professional. They can help determine the appropriate dosage based on individual needs and monitor for any potential side effects or interactions with other medications.

In summary, boron has been suggested to have anti-inflammatory properties that can reduce the symptoms of arthritis and improve joint health. Boron may help reduce inflammation by reducing levels of inflammatory markers in the blood and increasing levels of antioxidants in the body. However, the optimal dosage of boron for treating arthritis has not been established, and excessive boron intake can be toxic. Therefore, individuals who wish to supplement with boron for arthritis should do so under the guidance of a healthcare professional.

Boron and inflammatory bowel disease

Inflammatory bowel disease (IBD) is a chronic inflammatory condition that affects the digestive tract and can cause symptoms such as abdominal pain, diarrhea, and weight loss. Boron has been suggested to have anti-inflammatory properties that may help reduce inflammation in the digestive tract and improve symptoms of IBD.

Research has shown that boron supplementation can reduce levels of inflammatory markers in the blood, such as interleukin-6 (IL-6) and tumor necrosis factor alpha (TNF-alpha), which are commonly elevated in people with IBD. Boron may also help increase levels of antioxidants in the body, which can help reduce inflammation and protect the digestive tract from damage.

One study published in the journal Digestive Diseases and Sciences found that boron supplementation improved symptoms and reduced inflammation in patients with ulcerative colitis, a type of IBD. Another study published in the journal Biological Trace Element Research found that boron supplementation reduced inflammation in rats with colitis.

The recommended daily intake of boron for adults is 1-3 mg per day. However, the optimal dosage of boron for treating IBD has not been established. It is important to note that excessive boron intake can be toxic and may cause adverse effects such as nausea, vomiting, and diarrhea.

As a result, persons who wish to supplement with boron for IBD should do so under the supervision of a healthcare expert. They can assist in determining the proper dosage based on individual needs, as well as monitoring for any potential adverse effects or interactions with other medications.

In summary, boron has been shown to have anti-inflammatory characteristics that can reduce inflammation in the digestive tract and relieve symptoms of IBD. Boron may help reduce inflammation by reducing levels of inflammatory markers in the blood and raising levels of antioxidants in the body. However, the ideal dosage of boron for treating IBD has not been found, and excessive boron intake can be harmful. Hence, persons who seek to supplement with boron for IBD should do so under the advice of a healthcare professional.

Boron and allergies

Allergies are a common immune system response that can cause symptoms such as sneezing, itching, and inflammation. Boron has been suggested to have anti-allergic properties that may help reduce allergy symptoms and improve overall immune function.

Boron supplementation has been proven in studies to increase immune function by increasing levels of immunoglobulin antibodies, which are vital for combating infections and allergies. Boron may also aid in the reduction of inflammation in the body, which can exacerbate allergy symptoms.

Boron supplementation was observed to lessen the severity of allergy reactions in rats in one study published in the journal Biological Trace Element Research. Boron supplementation reduced inflammation in mice with allergic asthma, according to another study published in the journal Inflammatory Research.

The recommended daily intake of boron for adults is 1-3 mg per day. However, the optimal dosage of boron for treating allergies has not been established. It is important to note that excessive boron intake can be toxic and may cause adverse effects such as nausea, vomiting, and diarrhea.

Therefore, it is recommended that individuals who wish to supplement with boron for allergies do so under the guidance of a healthcare professional. They can help determine the appropriate dosage based on individual needs and monitor for any potential side effects or interactions with other medications.

Boron has been claimed to have anti-allergic properties that can alleviate allergy symptoms while also improving general immune function. Boron may promote immune function by increasing immunoglobulin antibody levels and decreasing inflammation in the body. However, the appropriate boron dosage for treating allergies has not been determined, and excessive boron consumption can be hazardous. Those who want to take boron supplements for allergies should do so under the supervision of a healthcare expert.

CHAPTER FOUR

Boron and Brain Function

The role of Boron in brain function

Boron is a mineral that plays a crucial role in the proper functioning of the human body. It has been suggested that boron may also have a positive impact on brain function.

Research has shown that boron plays a role in the formation and maintenance of neural connections in the brain. It may also improve cognitive function, memory, and attention span. Studies have also suggested that boron may have a neuroprotective effect, helping to protect brain cells from damage and reducing the risk of neurodegenerative diseases such as Alzheimer's and Parkinson's.

One study published in the journal Environmental Health Perspectives found that boron supplementation improved cognitive performance in older adults. Another study published in the journal

Nutritional Neuroscience found that boron supplementation improved cognitive function in healthy young adults.

The recommended daily intake of boron for adults is 1-3 mg per day. However, the optimal dosage of boron for improving brain function has not been established. It is important to note that excessive boron intake can be toxic and may cause adverse effects such as nausea, vomiting, and diarrhea.

Therefore, it is recommended that individuals who wish to supplement with boron for brain function do so under the guidance of a healthcare professional. They can help determine the appropriate dosage based on individual needs and monitor for any potential side effects or interactions with other medications.

In summary, boron plays a role in the formation and maintenance of neural connections in the brain and may improve cognitive function, memory, and attention span. Boron may also have a neuroprotective effect, helping to protect brain cells from damage and reducing the risk of neurodegenerative diseases. However, the optimal dosage of boron for improving brain function has not been established, and excessive boron intake can be toxic. Therefore, individuals who wish to supplement with boron for brain function should do so under the guidance of a healthcare professional.

Boron and memory

Boron is a mineral that is essential for optimal health and is involved in various physiological processes, including brain function and memory. While there is limited research on the effects of boron on memory, some studies have suggested that it may have a positive impact on cognitive function, which includes memory.

According to research it was found that boron supplementation improved short-term memory and concentration in healthy adults. Another study conducted on rats found that boron supplementation improved spatial memory and learning.

Furthermore, research suggests that boron may also be beneficial for individuals with memory-related diseases such as dementia and Alzheimer's disease. A study published in the Journal of Alzheimer's Disease found that boron supplementation improved cognitive function and reduced oxidative stress in individuals with mild cognitive impairment, a condition that often precedes dementia.

The recommended daily intake of boron for adults is 1-3 mg per day. However, the optimal dosage of boron for improving memory and memory-related diseases has not been established.

It is important to note that excessive boron intake can be toxic and may cause adverse effects such as nausea, vomiting, and diarrhea. Therefore, individuals who wish to supplement with boron for memory-related issues should do so under the guidance of a healthcare professional. They can help determine the appropriate dosage based on individual needs and monitor for any potential side effects or interactions with other medications.

In summary, while research on the relationship between boron and memory is limited, some studies suggest that boron supplementation may have a positive impact on cognitive function and memory. Boron may also be beneficial for individuals with memory-related diseases such as dementia and Alzheimer's disease. The recommended daily intake of boron for adults is 1-3 mg per day, but the optimal dosage for improving memory and memory-related diseases has not been established. Individuals who wish to supplement with boron for memory-related issues should do so under the guidance of a healthcare professional.

Boron and attention deficit hyperactivity disorder (ADHD)

Attention deficit hyperactivity disorder (ADHD) is a neurodevelopmental disorder that affects millions of children worldwide. Children with ADHD often have difficulties with attention, impulsivity, and hyperactivity, which can impact their academic and social functioning. While the exact causes of ADHD are not fully understood, some research suggests that nutrient deficiencies, including boron, may play a role.

Boron has been shown to improve brain function and cognitive ability, and some research suggest that boron supplementation may benefit youngsters with ADHD. Boron has been shown to boost dopamine levels in the brain, which is a crucial neurotransmitter for attention and focus. Furthermore, boron has been demonstrated to boost cognitive ability and memory, which may aid ADHD children.

Although research on the usefulness of boron supplementation for ADHD is limited, preliminary findings are promising. Boron supplementation improved attention, memory, and cognitive performance in children with ADHD, according to a study published in the Journal of Trace Elements in Medicine and Biology. Boron supplementation increased cognitive function and lowered hyperactivity in children with ADHD, according to another study published in the Journal of Child Neurology.

The dosage of boron for treating ADHD has not been established, but some studies have used doses ranging from 3 to 6 mg per day. It is important to note that boron supplementation should be done under the guidance of a healthcare professional, as high doses of boron can be toxic.

In conclusion, boron may be a promising natural supplement for children with ADHD. While further research is needed to fully understand its effectiveness and optimal dosage, preliminary studies have shown positive results. However, it is important to consult with a healthcare professional before starting any new supplement regimen for children with ADHD.

Boron and Menopausal Symptoms

Menopause is a natural biological process that occurs in women, usually between the ages of 45 and 55, marking the end of their reproductive years. During this period, women experience various symptoms, such as hot flashes, night sweats, vaginal dryness, mood swings, and reduced libido, which can significantly impact their quality of life. Boron has been studied for its potential to alleviate some of these symptoms.

Boron has been shown to increase the levels of estrogen in postmenopausal women, which can help alleviate symptoms such as hot flashes, night sweats, and vaginal dryness. Estrogen also plays a crucial role in maintaining bone health, and boron's ability to increase estrogen levels can help prevent osteoporosis, which is more common in postmenopausal women.

Boron has been shown to enhance levels of vitamin D and magnesium, which can improve bone density and lower the risk of fractures in addition to its effects on estrogen levels. Boron's capacity to raise magnesium levels can also aid in the relief of menopausal symptoms such as irritability and anxiety.

The amount of boron needed to relieve menopausal symptoms is unknown, but studies have shown that taking a daily supplement of 3 to 6 mg of boron can enhance estrogen levels and improve bone health. However, because high dosages of boron can be harmful, it is critical to see a healthcare expert before taking any boron supplements.

In conclusion, boron's ability to increase estrogen levels, vitamin D, and magnesium, makes it a promising natural supplement for alleviating menopausal symptoms and improving bone health. However, further research is required to determine the optimal dosage and long-term safety of boron supplementation.

Boron and hot flashes

Hot flashes are one of the most common and distressing symptoms of menopause. They are characterized by sudden and intense feelings of warmth, sweating, and flushing that can last for a few seconds to several minutes. Hot flashes can be triggered by a variety of factors, including stress, caffeine, alcohol, spicy foods, and hormonal imbalances.

Boron has been demonstrated to help menopausal women reduce the frequency and intensity of hot flashes. This is because boron aids in the regulation of estrogen and other hormone levels in the body. This can assist to reduce the hormonal abnormalities that might cause hot flashes.

Boron supplements have been shown in studies to considerably reduce the number of hot flashes experienced by menopausal women. In one study, women who took 3 mg of boron daily had 48% fewer hot flashes per day, compared to 31% less in women who received a placebo.

Boron is indicated at a dose of 3 mg per day to alleviate hot flashes. It should be noted, however, that boron supplements can interfere with some drugs, such as diuretics and blood thinners. As a result, it is critical to consult with your doctor before using boron supplements, especially if you are taking any drugs.

Overall, boron is a safe and effective natural remedy for menopausal hot flashes. It works by helping to regulate hormones in the body, which can reduce the frequency and severity of hot flashes. If you are experiencing hot flashes, talk to your healthcare provider about incorporating boron supplements into your treatment plan.

Boron and vaginal dryness

Vaginal dryness is a common symptom experienced by women during menopause. It occurs due to a decrease in the production of estrogen, which leads to a thinning and drying of the vaginal tissues. This can cause discomfort, itching, burning, and pain during sexual intercourse.

Boron has been shown to help alleviate vaginal dryness and restore vaginal moisture. It does so by increasing the levels of estrogen in the body, which in turn improves the health and lubrication of the vaginal tissues.

A study found that postmenopausal women who supplemented with boron for 8 weeks experienced a significant improvement in their vaginal health and moisture levels. The women in the study took 10 mg of boron daily.

Another study published in the Journal of Women's Health & Gender-Based Medicine found that boron supplementation helped alleviate vaginal dryness and other menopausal symptoms such as hot flashes, night sweats, and mood swings. The women in the study took 6 mg of boron daily.

It is important to note that boron supplementation should be done under the guidance of a healthcare professional, as excessive doses can have negative effects on the body. The recommended daily intake of boron for adults is 1-3 mg.

In addition to boron supplementation, other natural remedies that can help alleviate vaginal dryness include using a water-based lubricant during intercourse, staying hydrated, and practicing good hygiene. Women should also discuss their symptoms with their healthcare provider to determine the best course of treatment for their individual needs.

Boron and mood swings

Boron has been shown to have potential benefits in alleviating mood swings during menopause. As menopause can often lead to hormonal imbalances, it can result in irritability, anxiety, and depression. Boron can help regulate hormone levels, which in turn can improve mood swings.

A study conducted on postmenopausal women showed that boron supplementation significantly improved their mood scores. The participants were given a daily dose of 3mg of boron, and after four weeks, their mood had significantly improved.

Another study was conducted on male bodybuilders, where it was found that those who consumed boron supplements had significantly lower levels of depression compared to those who didn't consume the supplement.

The recommended dosage for boron supplementation varies depending on age, sex, and health conditions. The adequate intake of boron for adult men and women is around 1mg/day. However, studies have shown that doses of up to 10mg/day are safe and well-tolerated in healthy individuals.

It is important to note that boron supplementation should not replace traditional treatments for mood disorders, and individuals should always consult with a healthcare professional before starting any new supplement regimen.

Boron and Wound Healing

The role of Boron in wound healing

Boron has been found to play an important role in wound healing, both in terms of speeding up the healing process and reducing the risk of infection. This is due to its ability to increase the production of collagen, a protein that is essential for the formation of new tissue.

Collagen helps to provide structure to the skin and other tissues, and is also necessary for the formation of blood vessels. By increasing the production of collagen, boron can help to promote the growth of new tissue and blood vessels in and around the wound.

Boron also possesses antibacterial characteristics, which can aid in the prevention of wound infection. Furthermore, it has been demonstrated to have anti-inflammatory qualities, which can aid in the reduction of swelling and the promotion of healing.

Boron has been proven in studies to be useful in improving wound healing in a variety of diseases, including burns, surgical wounds, and diabetic foot ulcers. Boron supplementation dosage varies based on the severity of the wound and the individual's overall health, but typically ranges between 3-9mg per day.

It is worth noting that while boron supplementation can be beneficial for wound healing, it is not a replacement for proper wound care. In order to ensure optimal healing, it is important to keep the wound clean and protected, and to follow any other recommended treatment protocols as advised by a healthcare professional.

Boron and skin health

Boron is a trace element that plays an essential role in maintaining healthy skin. Its ability to support wound healing and tissue repair makes it a valuable nutrient for promoting healthy skin. Boron is believed to enhance the production of collagen, a protein that is essential for skin health. Collagen provides structure and elasticity to the skin and helps to maintain its youthful appearance. Boron also has anti-inflammatory properties that can help to reduce redness and swelling associated with skin conditions such as acne, eczema, and psoriasis.

Research has shown that boron supplementation can be effective in improving various skin conditions. In one study, boron supplementation was found to be effective in reducing the symptoms of psoriasis, a chronic inflammatory skin condition. The study showed that patients who took boron supplements experienced a significant improvement in their symptoms, including a reduction in redness, itching, and scaling.

In another study, boron supplementation was found to be effective in reducing the symptoms of acne, a common skin condition that is characterized by the formation of pimples, blackheads, and whiteheads. The study showed that participants who took boron supplements experienced a significant reduction in the number of pimples and blackheads on their skin.

Boron supplements are available in various forms, including capsules, tablets, and liquid formulations. The recommended dosage of boron supplements may vary depending on the specific skin condition being treated. However, a general dosage recommendation for boron supplementation is 3-6 mg per day.

While boron is a good vitamin for developing healthy skin, excessive boron consumption can be hazardous to health. Boron poisoning can result from high doses, causing symptoms such as nausea, vomiting, and diarrhea. As a result, before beginning boron supplementation, consult with a healthcare expert to identify the optimum dosage and ensure that it is safe for you to consume.

Boron and scar reduction

Boron has been found to have a beneficial effect on wound healing and scar reduction. It has been shown to stimulate cell proliferation and collagen synthesis, two important processes in wound healing and tissue repair. Additionally, it has anti-inflammatory properties that can reduce swelling and redness in the affected area.

Boron can be applied topically in the form of a cream or ointment. It can also be taken orally as a supplement. However, the dosage required for optimal wound healing and scar reduction is not yet clear and may vary depending on the severity of the wound or scar.

Studies have shown that boron supplementation can improve wound healing in animal models. In one study, rats with skin wounds were given boron supplementation for 14 days. The boron group showed significant improvement in wound healing compared to the control group.

In a different trial, a topical boron cream was used to treat individuals with surgical wounds. Compared to the control group, the cream considerably reduced the wound area's redness, edema, and pain.

Furthermore, scarring has been reported to be reduced by boron. Patients in a research on surgical scars received boron cream treatment for three months. Compared to the control group, the cream considerably decreased the size, redness, and hardness of the scars.

However, it is important to note that the dosage and duration of boron supplementation or topical application may vary depending on the individual and the severity of the wound or scar. It is recommended to consult a healthcare professional before starting any new supplement or topical treatment.

CHAPTER FIVE

Boron and Cancer

The role of Boron in cancer prevention

Due to its anti-inflammatory and anti-proliferative characteristics, it has been demonstrated that boron may have a role in the prevention of cancer. Boron has been proven to lower the body's levels of pro-inflammatory cytokines and chemokines, which have been linked to the onset and progression of cancer. Boron appears to also cause apoptosis, or planned cell death, which appears to slow the proliferation of cancer cells.

According to studies, boron supplements can lower the chance of developing some malignancies, such as breast, lung, and prostate cancer. According to one study, males who had greater blood levels of boron had a lower risk of developing prostate cancer. According to a different study, women who consumed more boron had a lower risk of developing breast cancer.

Boron also appears to have potential in cancer treatment. It has been shown to enhance the efficacy of chemotherapy drugs, possibly by increasing the uptake of the drugs into cancer cells. Boron neutron capture therapy (BNCT) is a form of radiation therapy that uses boron to selectively target cancer cells. In BNCT, boron is injected into the body, where it accumulates in cancer cells. The cells are then irradiated with neutrons, which react with the boron to produce high-energy alpha particles that selectively kill the cancer cells.

However, the optimal dosage of boron for cancer prevention and treatment is not yet clear. Further research is needed to determine the most effective doses and to fully understand the mechanisms by which boron acts to prevent and treat cancer. It is also important to note that boron should not be used as a replacement for conventional cancer treatments, but rather as a complementary therapy under the guidance of a healthcare professional.

Boron and breast cancer

Boron has been found to have a potential role in the prevention of breast cancer. Studies suggest that boron can inhibit the growth of breast cancer cells by inducing apoptosis, or programmed cell death, in these cells.

The dosage of boron required for breast cancer prevention is not well established. However, studies suggest that a daily intake of 3-6 mg of boron may help to reduce the risk of breast cancer. Foods that are rich in boron, such as nuts, dried fruits, and vegetables, can help to provide an adequate intake of this mineral.

It is important to note that boron should not be used as a standalone treatment for breast cancer. Instead, it should be used as a complementary therapy alongside conventional treatments such as chemotherapy and radiation therapy.

Boron has also been found to be effective in preventing other types of cancer such as prostate cancer, lung cancer, and cervical cancer. However, more research is needed to establish the exact dosage of boron required for cancer prevention and to determine its effectiveness as a standalone therapy.

Boron and prostate cancer

Boron has been studied extensively for its potential role in preventing and treating various types of cancer, including prostate cancer. Prostate cancer is a common type of cancer in men, and its incidence increases with age. It is important to note that boron is not a cure for prostate cancer, but it may have a role to play in preventing the development of this disease.

Studies have shown that boron may be effective in preventing the development of prostate cancer by inhibiting the growth of cancer cells. Boron has also been found to enhance the effectiveness of certain chemotherapy drugs used to treat prostate cancer, such as cisplatin.

The dosage of boron needed to effectively prevent or treat prostate cancer is not yet fully understood, as more research is needed to establish the optimal dose. However, it is generally recommended that adults consume around 3-5 mg of boron per day, which can be obtained through diet or supplementation.

To use boron to help prevent or treat prostate cancer, it is important to consult with a healthcare provider who can guide you in determining the appropriate dosage and provide guidance on potential interactions with other medications or health conditions. Additionally, it is important to maintain a healthy lifestyle by consuming a balanced diet rich in fruits, vegetables, and whole grains, exercising regularly, and avoiding smoking and excessive alcohol consumption, which can increase the risk of developing prostate cancer.

Potential Miracle Cure

The role of Boron and Pineal Gland

Melatonin, a small endocrine gland that is essential for regulating sleep-wake cycles, is produced and regulated by the pineal gland, a small organ situated deep inside the brain. Several scientists think that boron may be involved in the control of the pineal gland.

Research on the particular effects of boron on the pineal gland is few, but some studies have suggested that boron may boost melatonin production. Melatonin has been found to improve sleep quality and duration, reduce inflammation, and control immunological function, among other positive benefits on health.

Furthermore, some studies have suggested that melatonin may have anti-cancer properties and may help protect against other chronic diseases. Therefore, by supporting the pineal gland and promoting the production of melatonin, boron may help protect against certain diseases.

It is important to note that more research is needed to fully understand the relationship between boron and the pineal gland, as well as the potential health benefits of boron supplementation for pineal gland function.

Overall, while the role of boron in pineal gland function is still not fully understood, the potential health benefits of boron for other areas of health, such as bone health, hormone regulation, and cancer prevention, make it an important nutrient to consider adding to your diet or supplement routine.

Boron and Candida

Candida is a type of yeast that is naturally present in the human body. However, overgrowth of Candida can lead to various health problems, including fatigue, digestive issues, and even mood disorders. Boron has been found to be effective in inhibiting the growth of Candida.

Several studies have shown that boron can help in reducing the growth of Candida in the body. Boron can also help in reducing the symptoms associated with Candida overgrowth. The recommended dosage of boron for treating Candida is 3-9 mg per day.

Boron supplements can be taken orally in the form of capsules or tablets. Boron can also be obtained naturally from food sources such as almonds, peanuts, avocado, and apples.

It is important to note that while boron can be helpful in treating Candida, it should not be used as the sole treatment. A holistic approach that includes dietary changes and other natural remedies is necessary for effective treatment of Candida overgrowth. It is also important to consult with a healthcare provider before taking boron supplements to treat Candida or any other health condition.

Boron and Multiple Sclerosis

Multiple sclerosis (MS) is a chronic autoimmune disease that affects the central nervous system (CNS). It is characterized by the destruction of myelin, a fatty substance that surrounds and insulates nerve fibers, leading to impaired nerve signal transmission. Symptoms of MS include fatigue, muscle weakness, difficulty with coordination and balance, cognitive impairment, and vision problems.

Research suggests that boron may play a role in reducing inflammation and oxidative stress, both of which are implicated in the development and progression of MS. Boron may also support the regeneration of damaged myelin, as it has been shown to increase the activity of certain enzymes involved in myelin production.

A study published in the journal Biological Trace Element Research found that supplementation with boron significantly reduced the severity of symptoms in a group of MS patients. The study participants took 6 mg of boron per day for two months, after which their symptoms improved significantly compared to a control group.

Another study published in the Journal of Medicinal Food found that boron supplementation improved cognitive function and reduced oxidative stress in MS patients. The study participants took 6 mg of boron per day for four weeks.

While more research is needed to fully understand the role of boron in MS, these studies suggest that boron supplementation may be a safe and effective adjunct therapy for MS patients. It is important to note, however, that boron supplementation should be used in conjunction with conventional MS treatments, and should not be used as a replacement for these treatments.

The recommended dosage of boron for MS patients has not been established, and may vary depending on the individual. It is recommended that individuals consult with their healthcare provider before beginning any new supplement regimen, including boron supplementation for MS.

CHAPTER SIX

Detoxification with Boron

Boron has been shown to be effective in helping with detoxification processes in the body. One of the ways that boron aids in detoxification is by supporting the function of the liver, which is the primary organ responsible for filtering and eliminating toxins from the body.

Studies have shown that boron can help to protect the liver from damage caused by toxins such as alcohol and certain drugs. It does this by increasing the production of enzymes that help to detoxify the liver, and by reducing the formation of free radicals that can cause damage to liver cells.

In addition to its liver-protective effects, boron has also been shown to have chelating properties. This means that it can bind to heavy metals such as lead, mercury, and cadmium, and help to eliminate them from the body.

Boron has also been shown to support the function of the kidneys, which are responsible for filtering and eliminating waste products from the body. It does this by improving the efficiency of the kidneys in removing waste, and by reducing the formation of kidney stones.

To support detoxification, it is recommended to supplement with boron in a safe and appropriate dose. The recommended daily intake of boron for adults is 1-3 mg per day, although doses as high as 10 mg per day have been used in some studies without adverse effects.

It is important to note that while boron can be helpful in supporting detoxification processes, it should not be relied on as the sole method of detoxification. Eating a healthy diet, drinking plenty of water, getting regular exercise, and reducing exposure to toxins in the environment are also important factors in supporting overall detoxification and maintaining optimal health.

Effects of boron on viruses, bacteria, Fungi etc

Boron has been found to have antiviral, antibacterial, and antifungal properties, which make it a useful natural remedy for fighting infections. Here are some of the effects of boron on various pathogens:

- Viruses: Boron has been shown to inhibit the replication of some viruses, such as HIV, herpes simplex virus, and influenza virus. It does so by interfering with the virus's ability to attach to host cells and replicate.

- Bacteria: Boron has antibacterial properties and has been found to be effective against various strains of bacteria, including Staphylococcus aureus and Escherichia coli. It works by disrupting the bacterial cell wall and membrane, leading to cell death.

- Fungi: Boron has antifungal properties and has been found to be effective against various strains of fungi, including Candida albicans and Aspergillus niger. It works by disrupting the fungal cell wall and membrane, leading to cell death.

In addition to its direct effects on pathogens, boron has also been found to boost the immune system, which can help the body fight off infections more effectively.

However, it is important to note that while boron has demonstrated some antiviral, antibacterial, and antifungal properties, it should not be relied upon as the sole treatment for infections. Consult with a healthcare professional for proper diagnosis and treatment.

Quantity of boron the body needs at different ages

The amount of boron that the body needs varies depending on factors such as age, sex, and overall health status. According to the National Institutes of Health (NIH), the recommended daily allowance (RDA) for boron is as follows:

- Infants 0-6 months: 0.2 milligrams (mg) per day
- Infants 7-12 months: 0.5 mg per day
- Children 1-3 years: 1 mg per day
- Children 4-8 years: 1.5 mg per day
- Children 9-13 years: 2 mg per day
- Adolescents 14-18 years: 3 mg per day
- Adults 19-50 years: 3 mg per day
- Adults 51 years and older: 3.5 mg per day
- Pregnant and lactating women: 3 mg per day

It is important to note that these are general recommendations, and the specific needs of an individual may vary. In addition, certain health conditions, such as osteoporosis or arthritis, may require higher doses of boron for optimal health benefits. However, it is important to talk to a healthcare provider before taking any supplements, especially at high doses.

Overall, it is essential to consume a balanced diet rich in boron-containing foods to ensure adequate intake of this important mineral. Good dietary sources of boron include fruits, vegetables, nuts, legumes, and whole grains. Some examples of boron-rich foods include avocados, almonds, hazelnuts, broccoli, oranges, grapes, and raisins.

CHAPTER SEVEN

Diet recipes that has boron intake and are healthy

While there is no specific diet or recipe that is tailored for high boron intake, incorporating certain foods in your diet can help increase your boron intake. Here are some healthy recipe ideas that contain foods high in boron:

Quinoa Salad with Chickpeas and Avocado

Ingredients:

- 1 cup quinoa
- 1 can chickpeas, drained and rinsed
- 1 avocado, diced
- 1 red bell pepper, diced
- 1/4 cup chopped fresh cilantro
- 2 tablespoons olive oil
- 2 tablespoons apple cider vinegar
- 1 teaspoon honey

- Salt and pepper to taste

Instructions:

1. Cook the quinoa according to package instructions.
2. In a large bowl, combine the cooked quinoa, chickpeas, avocado, red bell pepper, and cilantro.
3. In a small bowl, whisk together the olive oil, apple cider vinegar, honey, salt, and pepper.
4. Pour the dressing over the quinoa salad and toss to combine.
5. Serve immediately or store in the fridge for later.

Roasted Vegetables with Garlic and Herbs

Ingredients:

- 1 small butternut squash, peeled and diced
- 1 large sweet potato, peeled and diced

- 1 large red onion, sliced
- 2 garlic cloves, minced
- 2 tablespoons olive oil
- 1 tablespoon fresh rosemary, chopped
- 1 tablespoon fresh thyme, chopped
- Salt and pepper to taste

Instructions:

1. Preheat the oven to 400°F.
2. In a large bowl, toss together the butternut squash, sweet potato, red onion, garlic, olive oil, rosemary, thyme, salt, and pepper.
3. Spread the vegetables out in a single layer on a baking sheet.
4. Roast for 30-40 minutes, or until the vegetables are tender and golden brown.
5. Serve immediately or store in the fridge for later.

Salmon and Broccoli Stir-Fry

Ingredients:

- 1 pound salmon fillets, skin removed and cut into small pieces
- 1 head broccoli, cut into small florets
- 2 garlic cloves, minced
- 1 tablespoon fresh ginger, grated
- 2 tablespoons olive oil
- 2 tablespoons soy sauce
- 1 tablespoon honey
- 1 tablespoon cornstarch
- 1/4 cup water
- Salt and pepper to taste

Instructions:

1. In a small bowl, whisk together the soy sauce, honey, cornstarch, water, salt, and pepper.
2. Heat the olive oil in a large skillet over medium-high heat.

3. Add the salmon to the skillet and cook for 3-4 minutes on each side, or until cooked through.

4. Remove the salmon from the skillet and set aside.

5. Add the broccoli, garlic, and ginger to the skillet and cook for 3-4 minutes, or until the broccoli is tender-crisp.

6. Return the salmon to the skillet and pour the soy sauce mixture over the top.

7. Cook for an additional 1-2 minutes, or until the sauce has thickened.

8. Serve immediately over rice or noodles.

Where boron can be found

Boron can be found in a variety of food sources, including:

- Avocado
- Almonds
- Brazil nuts
- Raisins
- Prunes
- Peanut butter
- Lentils
- Chickpeas
- Beans (navy, kidney, and black)
- Broccoli
- Spinach
- Oranges
- Grapes
- Apples
- Pears

Boron supplements are also available in the US and can be purchased at health food stores, pharmacies, and online retailers. It's important to choose a reputable brand and to follow the recommended dosage instructions. Some popular boron supplements include:

- Solgar Boron 3mg
- Pure Encapsulations Boron Glycinate 2mg
- Country Life Boron 3mg
- NOW Foods Boron 3mg
- Nature's Life Boron 3mg

It's important to note that while boron supplements can be helpful in meeting daily intake requirements, it's always best to obtain nutrients through a well-rounded, nutrient-dense diet. If you have any concerns about your boron intake or wish to supplement, it's recommended to consult with a healthcare professional.

Boron Deficiency

Boron is an essential mineral that is required by the body in small amounts for various physiological functions. Boron deficiency occurs when the body doesn't get an adequate amount of boron from the diet or is unable to absorb or utilize it effectively. The deficiency of boron is a rare condition as boron is naturally present in most foods in small quantities. However, certain factors can contribute to boron deficiency, including low dietary intake, poor absorption, and excessive excretion.

One of the significant factors contributing to boron deficiency is low dietary intake. People who follow a diet that is low in fruits, vegetables, and nuts are at higher risk of developing boron deficiency. This is because these foods are rich sources of boron, and not consuming them regularly can lead to insufficient boron intake.

Another factor that can lead to boron deficiency is poor absorption of boron in the body. This can occur due to several reasons, including gastrointestinal disorders, malabsorption syndromes, and the use of certain medications that interfere with boron absorption.

Excessive excretion of boron from the body can also cause boron deficiency. This can happen due to excessive sweating, frequent urination, and the use of certain medications that promote boron excretion from the body.

Boron deficiency can lead to several health problems, including poor bone health, impaired brain function, reduced immune function, and hormonal imbalances. The symptoms of boron deficiency are not specific and can vary from person to person. owever, some of the common symptoms include joint pain, muscle weakness, fatigue, poor concentration, and memory problems.

The treatment of boron deficiency involves increasing boron intake through dietary changes or supplementation. Boron supplements are available in the form of capsules, tablets, and liquids. The dosage of boron supplements depends on the severity of the deficiency and the age of the individual. It is recommended to consult a healthcare professional before taking any boron supplements.

CONCLUSION

In conclusion, boron deficiency is a rare condition that can occur due to low dietary intake, poor absorption, and excessive excretion. It can lead to several health problems, and early diagnosis and treatment are essential to prevent further complications. Eating a balanced diet that includes fruits, vegetables, and nuts can help prevent boron deficiency. In case of deficiency, taking boron supplements can help restore the body's boron levels and improve overall health.

In conclusion, boron is a vital mineral that plays an essential role in maintaining overall health and wellbeing. From boosting bone health to reducing inflammation, improving brain function, and fighting cancer, boron has proven to be a miracle cure for many ailments.

While it is naturally present in various foods, some individuals may still experience boron deficiencies due to poor dietary habits or underlying health conditions. The symptoms of boron deficiencies are diverse and may range from poor memory and concentration to brittle bones, arthritis, and reduced fertility.

However, it is essential to note that excessive boron intake can also be harmful and may cause adverse effects such as nausea, vomiting, and diarrhea. Therefore, it is crucial to follow the recommended daily dosage of boron and avoid taking supplements without consulting a healthcare professional.

When it comes to taking boron supplements, it is crucial to purchase them from reputable sources and follow the recommended dosage carefully. It is also essential to consider the potential side effects, interactions with other medications, and allergies before taking boron supplements.

In summary, while boron has many potential health benefits, it is essential to approach its consumption with caution and mindfulness. By incorporating boron-rich foods into your diet, taking supplements under the guidance of a healthcare professional, and being mindful of dosage and potential side effects, you can enjoy the many health benefits that boron has to offer.

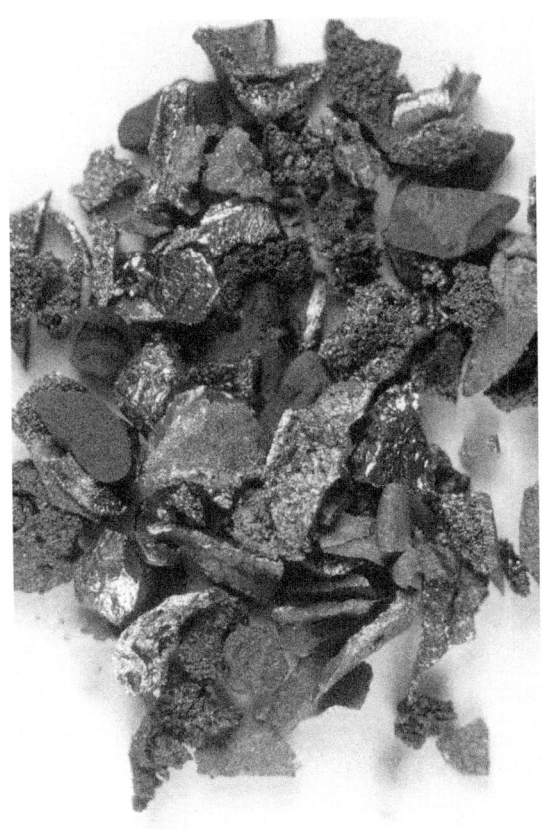

Printed in Great Britain
by Amazon

33087075R00066